MAY THE ANGE[illegible] S

POEMS OF LIFE, LOVE, AIDS & DEATH

By Mark and Andrew Peters

Our revels are now ended. These our actors
As I foretold you, were all spirits, and
Are melted into air, into thin air:
And like the baseless fabric of this vision,
The cloud-capp'd towers, the gorgeous palaces,
The solemn temples, the great globe itself,
Yea, all which it inherit shall dissolve,
And like this insubstantial pageant faded,
Leave not a rack behind. We are such stuff
as dreams are made on: and our little life
Is rounded with a sleep

The Tempest,
William Shakespeare.

SHROPSHIRE EDUCATION SERVICES

SHROPSHIRE COUNTY COUNCIL

Shropshire Education Publications
The Shirehall, Abbey Foregate, Shrewsbury SY2 6ND Telephone 0743 254321
All profits from this book go to the Shrewsbury and Mid Wales Hospice

ISBN 1 899646 00

Acknowledgments

This book is dedicated to my mother, who has been through so much. Special thanks to Tim for his hard work and confidence in the project, and to Bruce Barr for helping me find my way. Thanks also to Nick and Liz at Legend who made the vision visible, and to Polly for her support and her sharp editorial eye.

Previous Publication of these poems

Andrew Peters:

'On Seeing My Brother's Body Lying In His Bed,' 'The Year Is Falling Now,' 'A Child's Poem' first appeared in *Heart Throb* (WM Arts literature magazine) 1994
'High Up In The Hills' first published in *Jugular Defences* (The Oscar's Press) 1994
'A Child's Poem,' 'My Brother's Snoring' have also been recorded for BBC Radio 4's *Talking Poetry* Programme 1994.

Mark Peters:

'The Seed' first published in *The Alegheny Review* (a National Journal of Undergraduate Literature) 1986
'Hyaa!' first appeared in *Secret Surrealist Society* 1990
Various of these poems appeared in *American Literary* (the arts and literary journal of the American University) and also in his first collection *'The Angel Parade'* (INRI Productions) 1993.

Contents

Preface	*page 1*
Acknowledgments	*page 2*
Previous publication	*page 2*
Introduction	*page 4*
From the funeral, a friend speaks	*page 5*
Part one - Childhood	*page 7*
Part two - Illness	*page 21*
Part three - Death	*page 49*
Part four - Reflections	*page 67*
Part five - Resolution	*page 85*
Biographies	*page 100*
Index	*page 102*

Introduction

When my brother first died, I did not know what to do with the grief. It was such a shock. I couldn't quite believe that he was dead and kept expecting him to ring up. People around me reacted in different ways. Some were loving and supportive. Others couldn't handle it. Death was a heavy subject which they had to change. My grief was so big that no one person could carry it for me. I had to do something with the feelings, had to find some way to make visible what lay unspoken inside.

And so I wrote and in writing, fell in love with this craft of poetry in a new and sad way. I experimented with sonnet, syllabic poem, blank verse and villanelle. They were houses to shelter my grief, words that became one half of this book.

In his will, Mark left me his diaries and poems. I cried so much reading them, and smiled at memories only we knew. Here was the brother I grew up with, loved and hated, feared and respected in equal measure. And here also was another man I had only been acquainted with - a writer with oceans of thought, lyrical, original, a true poet. I had always known Mark as a poet and we were too often competitive about our writing. But as I read his life and edited his poems, I wish I could have had time to tell him how much I admired his craftsmanship.Why did he have to die to make me see what jewels he carried?

Andrew Peters
September 1994

From the Funeral, a Friend Speaks

"I met Mark in 1985 at American University, and was completely overwhelmed, first by his beauty, I have to admit. And then, his nature. And then his poetry. He was the editor of the literary magazine at AU and he was the first person to publish my poetry, and we did not become close friends until May {1993} and then together, we worked feverishly on getting the Angel Parade out. (His first collection.) We worked really hard and sometimes we got stuck on details, but I swear to God, he was hanging on for this book. He said, "I want to hand my book to my mom, and to my brother, and to my friends." And Wednesday night, a couple of nights ago, I got it from the printer and I brought it over, and he was in a state where we didn't know if he was really there any more, but a bunch of us were round his bed, and we put flowers on his bed, and he opened his eyes. We hadn't seen him for days, because he would fade in and out. And he opened his eyes and looked at me and he went, "Oh yeah!" And I knew it was Mark, and I showed him his book, and I said, "I love you," and he said it back in his throat.

This for me was the moment....

Sylvana

Part One

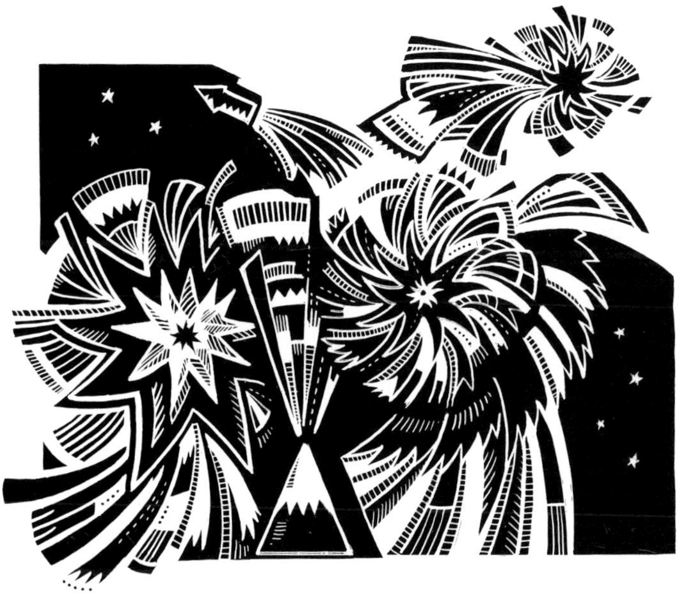

CHILDHOOD

The Gift

I was ten, you fourteen, adolescent:
Filled with living words, you sent me poems
From your far off school. How much they meant....
My Poet Brother! If there were exams
For showing off, I passed, proud, then grew
Into a stand-up man, poet too, loud:
Was heard, began to make a living, still do
While you, now scholar, shining in the crowd.

Your job then turned to Editor-In-Chief,
Honing words, the thrust of cut and paste:
Came AIDS to duel, thrust, cut and waste
And now I am your Editor-In-Grief
This death, a death-day gift you sent to me,
Your last breath spent, inspired my poetry.

A.P.

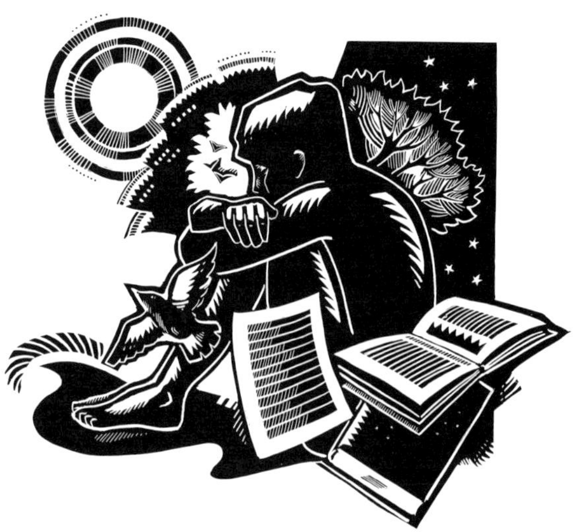

The Fair On Hampstead Heath

Coconuts!
Co-co nuts!
Come and get
your ***co-conuts!***

Here at the fairground
with the boys,
where the lights are
red and orange and yellow,
O... O... a holiday on
Hampstead Heath!

Boys wear green socks,
grey shirts, scout shorts,
all unlearned
how clouds are made
how knots are tied
how tents are staked.

Out of the barrel roll all
adults
out of the Rotor,
the spinning motor,
tumble-jumble
of lost keys, stop please!
feet off the ground.

By the ponds,
with their slimy fronds
sing frogs, bark dogs;
now down by the old log
old Jack sits,
he knows stories,
he's seen glories,
wars full of them,
two of them,
he don't worry.

Old tramp Jack,
with his two degrees,
with his old blue knees.
Cardboard Jack,
hard-up Jack,
wears a medallion on
his forehead,
like the sun,
he winks,
you know.

Me and the boys,
boyscouts one and two
and three and four
watch the birds and smoke cigars.
I've got money,
you've got money,
we've got money
to ride the rides:
the Caterpillar,
the Swing-Me-Round-Again,
the Wheel,
now don't fall out!

O the shyster stalls
and goldfish,
come on, throw the ball
now don't walk by;
you'll win, all win,
see what I told you,
here's a goldfish,
twofish,
threefish,
one for your mum,
now don't be shy.

Round the wheel goes,
round and round
and speakers and sound
and the trees and the
ground
and the breeze
and we stop,
just one more time
please,
one more time,
O make it stop!

M.P.

Guy Fawkes Night, Primrose Hill

Wind and rain,
What a pain!
Hot dogs,
Burning logs
I've got fags,
I'm full of blags

Spin the bottle!
Got any bottle?
Don't miss out,
Kissing's in
I want to *shout!*

Brother's got a girl,
She's put me in a whirl
I'm dead proud!
One of the crowd!
Spinning stops
Now's your chance
Lungs fill,
I will! I will!
Tongues dance....

Wow!
Now fireworks burst!
Thirst to be grown up,
Drunk on life
And flown up
Into the sky
Rockets!
Shock, it's
Catherine Wheels!
And Pyramids!
Bangers
Too quiet by half
Laugh,
Look up!
The sky is sprinkled with light
O... O... bright-a-bright night
On Primrose Hill.

A.P.

My Brother's Snoring

My brother's snoring
makes such a sound,
it shakes the bed
and shivers the ground.

I never get any sleep
Not even a peep,
because of that creep.

So,
I stick my two big toes
right up his nose!
It's the best way to stop him I've found!

A.P.

It All Happens Here

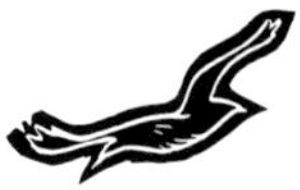

Shrieking birds clear paths
through woods I walk in,
echo in the mammoth vasts
a brotherhood of flames,
of tiny voices in a land of giants.

memories of children
fill with song the quantuum fields.

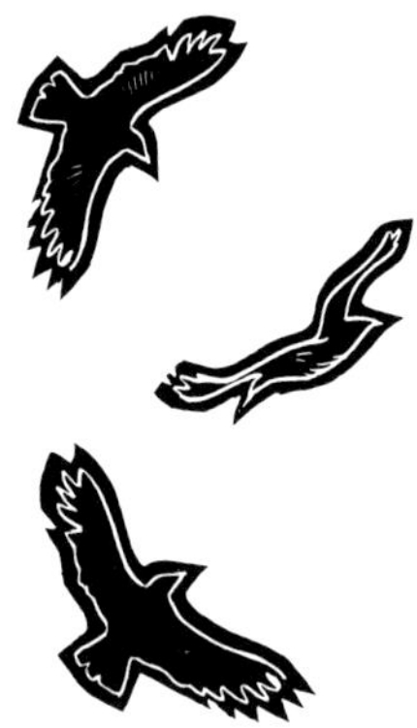

The mind that thinks the soul,
erects the son;
such life,
such burning life,
such crippling, brilliant life
the body cannot muffle,
staunch, nor dam,

memories of children
fill with song the quantuum fields.

And all to happen now,
My God ...
I cannot block my ears,
nor seal my eyes,
nor hold my mouth,
nor touch, nor sense
but Am, and am this self
no never again,

memories of children
fill with song the quantuum fields.

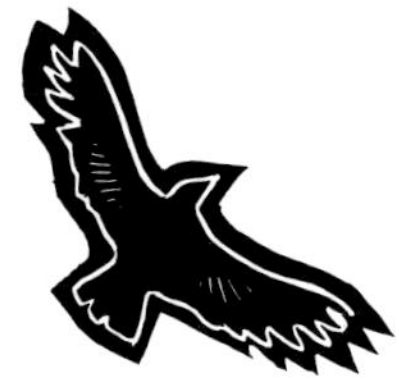

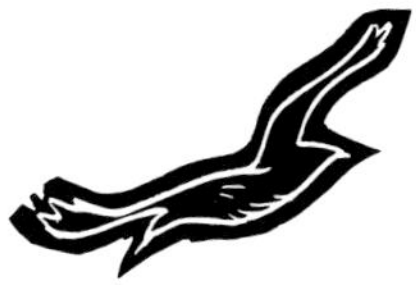

For this do lovers
ride the river's current,
for this the White Feet
set upon the sudden waters,
for this the Strife
to breach the ice-grey summits,
for this the Crimes, the Journeys,
Bloods, Acts, Poetries,
for this the All,
this tumbling Wave,

memories of children
fill with song the quantuum fields.

M.P.

The Burning Of Stubble

Two children leap
across golden, smoking
snakes of straw
that smoulder, burst
into orange dance.

Ben is pleased
his grain in the hops,
bare ground ready soon
for November's tilling,
tractor heaving against
a hard morning.

Two children hold hands
as the smoking snake's tail,
the slow river,
and swan feathers drift by
white as snow.

Now I'm sitting on 14th Street
watching dust on my boots,
the rain falling on them;
smoke from an English field
is in my nose,
swans, pale as ice, glide by,
dust turns to mud,
and it keeps raining.
Seasons seem to be changing.

M.P.

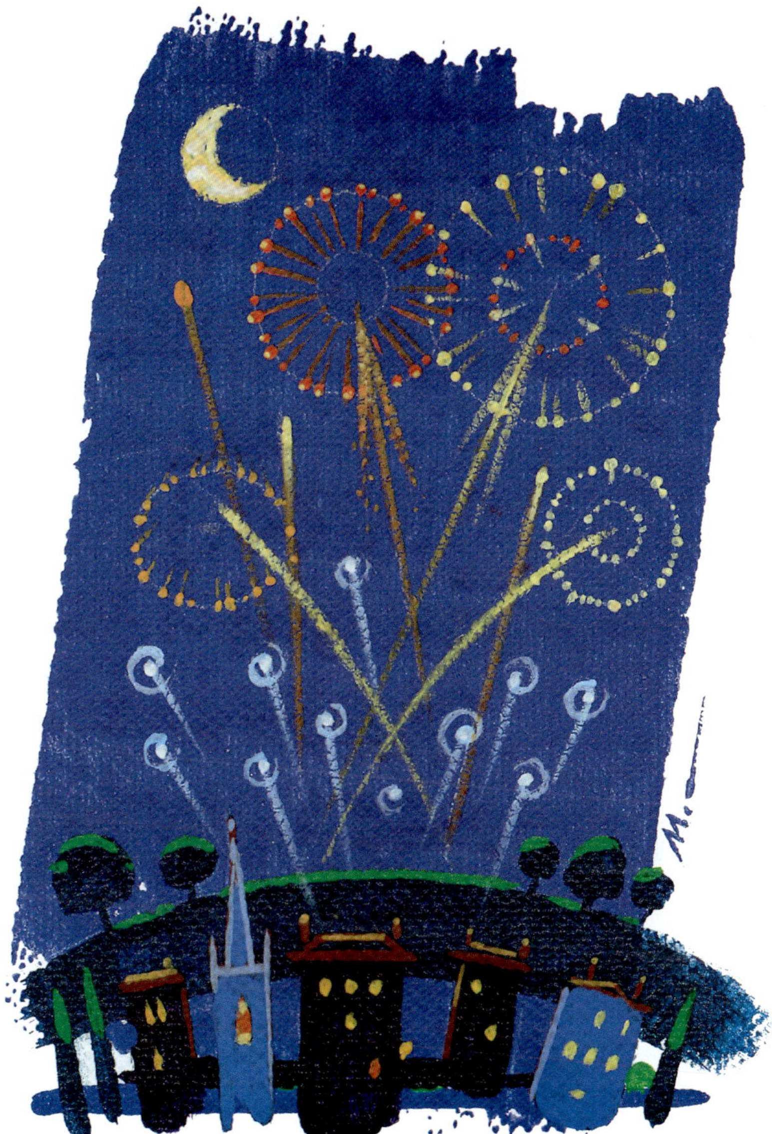

Guy Fawkes Night, Primrose Hill

Michael Ogden

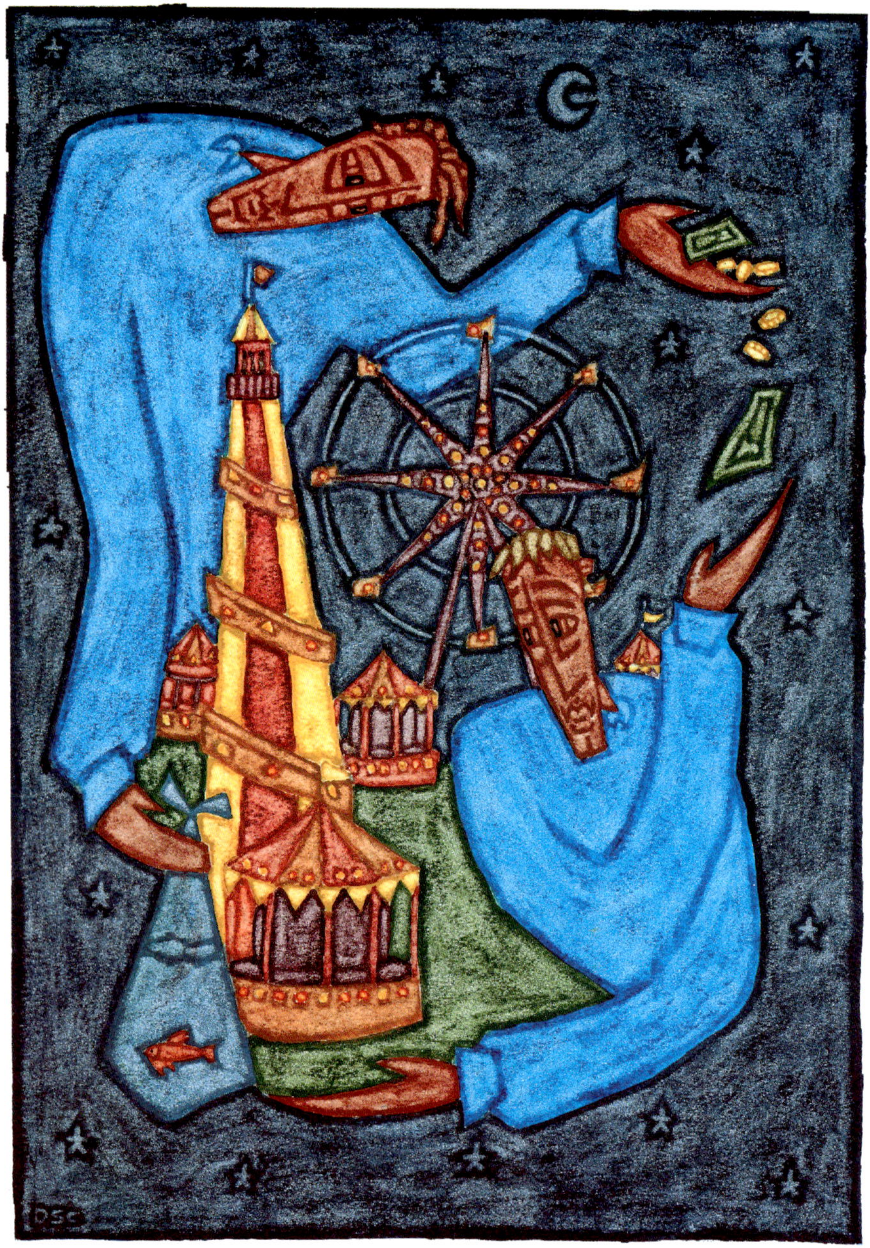

The Fair on Hampstead Heath

Dianne Cartwright

Child Song

I am littler than
the littlest ant
though the sun has
lit in my heart.

I am quieter than
the quietest mouse
though I have witnessed
the birth of man.

I am lighter than
the lightest weight
I have lost
but I've gained
I am born again.

I am softer than
my darling's voice
and this little, quiet
light, soft heart
has found its peace
and makes no noise.

M.P.

A Child's Poem

Why is there rain, and where does it come from mum?
And how come clouds live up in the sky?
And why did my brother get ill and die?

The rain is a river of tears, my dear,
For every cloud sees how sad we are here.
Yet I don't know why your brother should die.

Why are the leaves so bright and so green mum
And how do they learn to fall off and fly?
And why did my brother get ill and die?

Leaves are alive and filled with breath, my child.
At the end of the year, they have their death.
But I just don't know how my son could die.

And will he ever come back again mum?
And can't we find him if we really try?
And I'm so unhappy mum, why did he die?

He's taken a boat to the river of tears
And we shall not see him for so many years
So hold my hand, little one, and wave him goodbye.
So hold my hand tight, little one, and wave him goodbye.

A.P.

Part Two

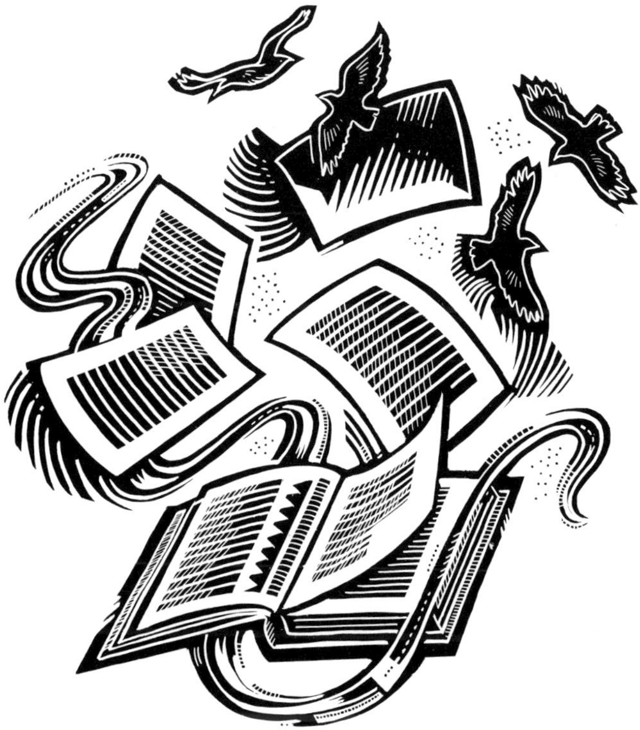

ILLNESS

Washington DC, Spring 1993

My brother lies on his bed in his room.
The bed is his room, his life.
He no longer understands the verb 'to get up'.
And outside, it rains a warm, spring rain,
making all the city shine into the night.
The peace here in this dying room is immense.
The walls cannot compete.
Instead, this quiet is given into the earth,
as my brother so soon shall be.

A child, a thirty-two year old child,
curled up, hugging the duvet,
drifting gently into and out of this roaring life.
Sleep, sleep shall be nice.
To rest would be a great thing for him.
Now his days,
his poet-days
are come this smallness,
this perfect smallness:
food, medication, rest, peeing.
It is so simple, a simplicity we all want.
No cares, except who to give his books to.

Oh! The car needs to be repaired, the bike too -
both great machines he will never sit in again:
but little travelling threads he hangs onto
so thin, so thin.
They are not delusions,
just a sorting of loose ends.

This roaring man.
His lust was frowned on by me,
the righteous brother.
And now, no lust, just the eyes of a boy,
looking out from a face that is not rosy
nor full-cheeked,
but filled with hollow places.
We won't walk in tall hills anymore,
nor ski, nor swear at the blisters on our feet,
nor try to out-run, out-poet, out-fame each other.

Now, our only yardstick is love.

A.P.

The Flame

The anvil has been struck
and the falling fires of trees
blind me, groping through November;
the sometimes hushed,
sometimes harsh
tinkle of a tiny stream
wends its way through Rock Creek,
through woods,
under this decrepit bridge,
its moss-rotten lumber.

O how the woods call me now,
O how the spirits are
in sudden masses all here ...
open-armed, the trees, the birds,
the whispering of frost-dried bracken -
immutable, impermeable silence
of cracked earth underfoot;

bless the flame that life is.

M.P.

My Soft Heartbeat

Our old windows
make the day outside look shallow,
from my bed
the room seems to expand,
beams and pine floor planks
sing to each other,
as the tap of rain
adds kisses.
I am silent,
for my body is a perfect thing.
Smoothly mechanic,
it makes no noise,
my soft heartbeat
could not scare a mouse.

M.P.

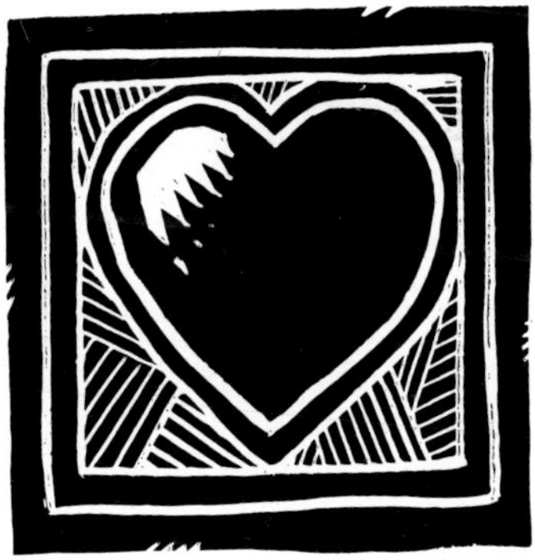

The Seed (For My Father)

Land locks her hold on the broiling molt,
the gilt smile of the cloudy bothered moon,
we reflect that earth has no hold,
none at all; the beaches shudder,
day is done.
Mahogany, elms, oak, the bark
that dreams itself into night, all one wood black;
like coalfires the seabirds circle in the dark.

There floats in the ragged drugged bier
of the water, your soul's ash,
calling the last letters of a far off youth,
reflected against the hard sepia of the far off sky;
writing in stuttering vermillions,
our sadness.

White broken beads of bone pearl,
like necklaces of flowers, wash up,
bearing blacker seeds than sun has known.
Harder breaths and hotter tears we have not shed,
arguing with a sudden night.

Under our feet the sea is speaking
a pulse for even a beatless heart;
often by the breakers scudding, dripping,
we now meditate, spirits rolling
endlessly in motion, falling-rising
in the swell that moves you still.

For you were the warm light in our warm house,
the comfort behind misty panes; bringing
like a hard sequoia, solidness, softness to our lives.
When the cold sounds of steel mills
woke us with their arguing,
and the sun moved where it chose,
when stars like fistfuls of granite
flung themselves against the glass,
we were safe.

Then, in the calm of all things,
the long lawns bordering roses in Hildesheim,
you heaved great white lungfuls
as snows fell on the children by the hill
sudden in their oranges and yellows,
poised in infinite flight;
poised at the pond's mirrored edge,
raw faces laughing and laughing.

By the water's yellow edge we sat
by palms, a Californian sun,
and now, years later, we say goodbye.
Then why did you die?
Letting life overboil, overcook, run dry;
spilling your body into dark degeneration,
your soul into the coma of God.
What hard bludgeon, what lucid harrowing
was the dream that took you to sleep?

The cedar forest, the elm and willow
shaded all of what your world was.
In the lush, open meadows
children peered through cracks in their fingers
at red, round strawberries;
in the coiling ornamental ponds of Regents Park,
how many wild birds!
even in the leaf-meal was life!

Now water's countless epitaphs in flaming
whites are flung up - bold, harsh songs,
crooning spirituals,
the centuries' repertoires.
All voices are here, and angelic choirs,
and the low fiend's moan;
Atlantis greets a friend.

And in our lives, we do not
speak too much anymore;
these witless waters foment disturbance,
the clouds rearing like our hopes run through
with steel, scattered like the tossed patterns
ashes make,
beneath our feet now.

Rock then in your safer home
where light won't sear your eyes or burn;
in the mumbling currents of icy seas,
rest in the pallor of dumb, blind ease,
foregoing life,
time, festivities and family.
We trail behind, bent at the border.

M.P.

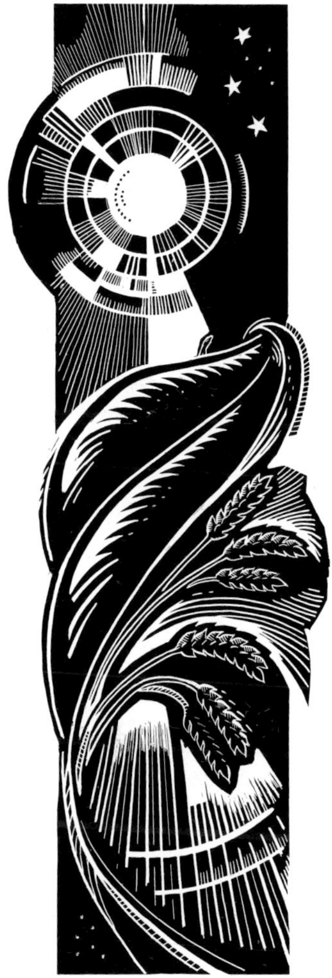

Autumn Spirits

Life has buried itself in old brown nuts
lying with the purple blood-worm
the sodden leaf,
and sleighbell bulbs stretch deep unwoken.

Life has left the house
stuffing its cheeks with flakes of sun, oaks,
the hunter waits.

A small spirit has risen dressed in gold;
she has danced for me,
danced in earth
that I have held my face to,
breathed into.

A spirit has parted the trees
and the green rain is singing,
singing and slapping,
and the bird is not in its nest,
but listening, above the ground.

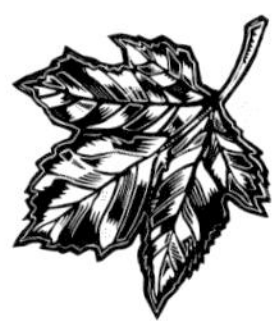

I sit in mud, cross-legged,
fresh mud, it smells in my cupped hands
like an Indian prayer;
I breathe in once, twice, three times,
the winter sky my mantle,
my soul a white feather
on a white swan's back,
a bloody snow eagle's.

M.P.

The Illness

I am not stricken with plague, scurvy, smallpox.
I am loaded with a life well lived.

When the microphone of Peter
is lifted to my lips
I'll say it was all worthwhile,
all, and nothing less.

Then, dare the being say my life was no life at all,
but sand, a test-tube experiment,
a mix of vapour, fluid, metal.

The architect of life has designed death also
and my mother will assure me as I go -
bones, blood, eyes, ears becoming formless-
my mother who played guitar to me and scratched my back,
my brother who I mistreated,
my father who I never understood,
what do I know of death?
What do I know of this loss,
except that I do not want to say goodbye...

Perhaps,
I'll carry a little memory like a drop of rain,
a green, curled leaf.
then, to be with angels and relatives
to sing and groan with the countless animals
that fill full the turning wheel's greatest circumference.

M.P.

A Time Of Year

i Acorns pop like mines
blister in the cool thin air,
smelling of rain.

ii *My new red heart*
is working well,
he says.

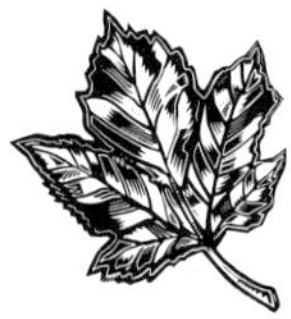

iii Although it isn't raining,
her feathers pour down
as she beats her breast
on the wire mesh.

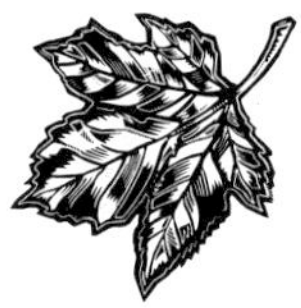

iv He smiles because of his years,
his cheeks like sharkskin.

v This year, acorns
drop like gunfire
on our green porch roof.

vi Children rush into the trees,
pull bracken and bramble
over themselves, showing
lionshead yellows through the
curl and coil of dead leaves,
sunflowers, leaving pink trails
under dripping saps, magnolia petals,
then their mouths grow thick,
bark, then wood,
Roddy, Graham, Adam, Esther,
Rosamund, Cairn, Simon, Petrus.

vii A cormorant stretches,
an oily blackbird,
I break the golden manna,
watch his neck plunge.

viii *I am ready,*
he says.

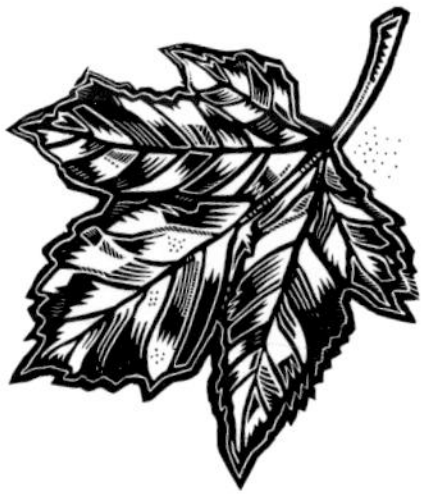

ix The oak leaves
like fallen feathers
are restless in
the rising wind,
the sky.

M.P.

Horse Of Night

Horse of my blackest addiction,
I have felt your blood race
the quarter mile between
my head and my heart,
and I have cheered you on,
and died at the starting gate,
and run with you,
with my heart in my mouth,
my whole body
miles down the road,

and I have collapsed,
spent, at the broken gate
you crossed
to gain your freedom,
and you dragged me on,
on a race no-one could win,
racing for racing's sake,
racing until your hard, proud,
black veins pumped dry,
and the sun
and moon
bowed to your hard body,

and today is tomorrow
and I am racing still.

M.P.

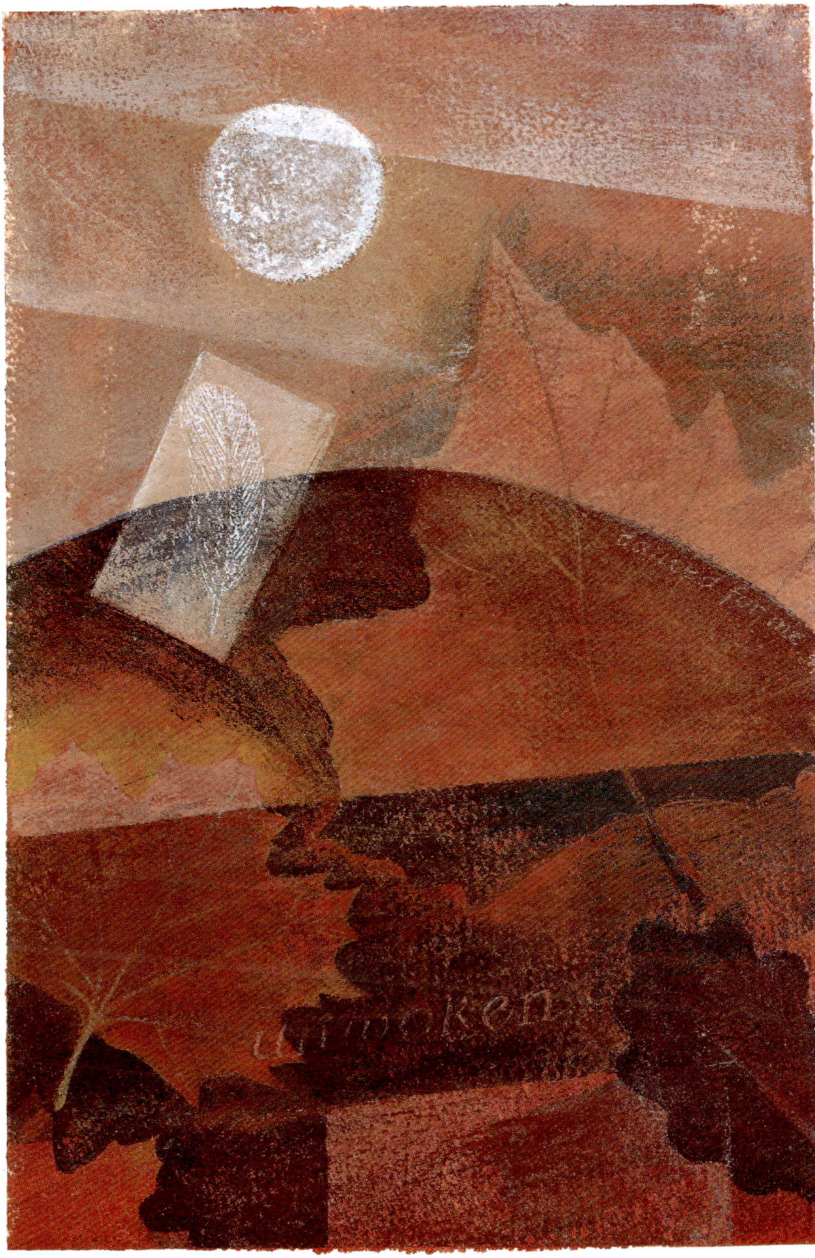

Autumn Spirits

Adrian Barclay

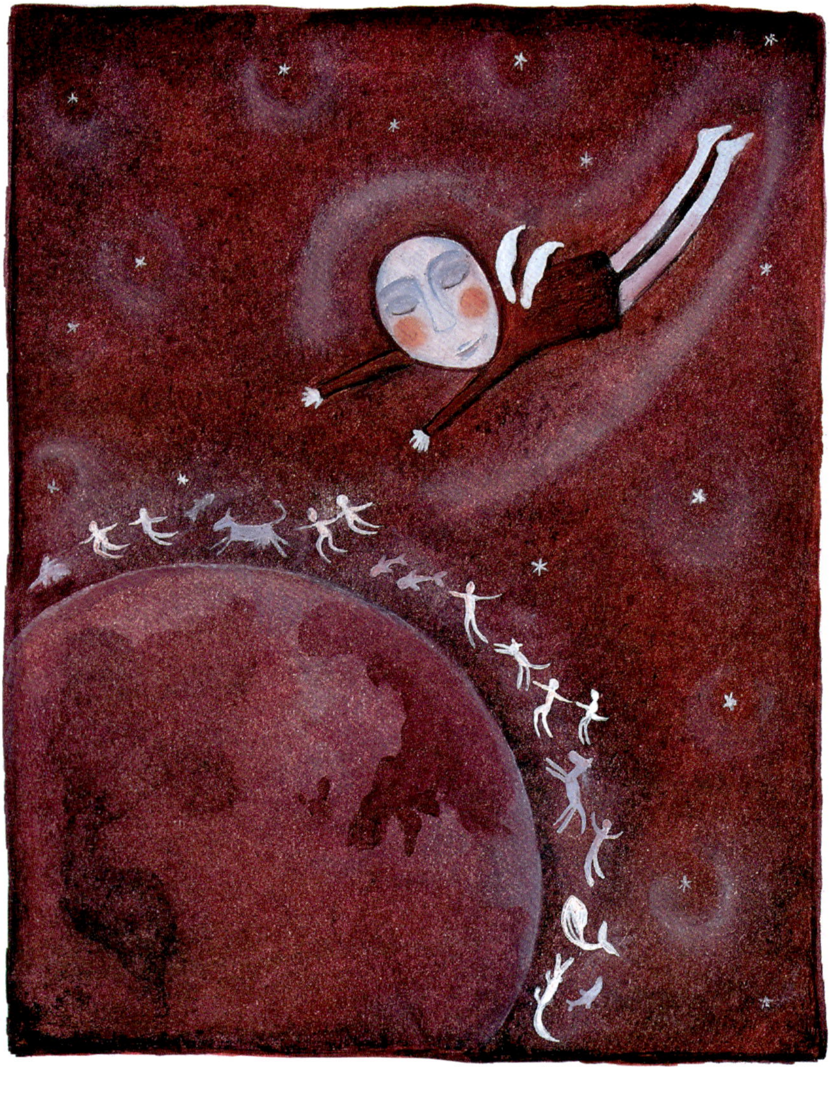

The Illness

Liz Marshall

The Dance Is Begun

Morphine was my answer
to the problem of motion,
a psychological travel-sickness
medication,
thinner to the rich oil palette,
verdünner to the
hard yellow sunflower's laugh.

It was the answer to morning,
cracking like an unripe egg,
the stretched out birth
with lungs too full of blood
to laugh,
with night too soon and cold,
too short, too fast,
the dream not yet begun
yet almost done.

M.P.

High Up In The Hills

High up in the hills,
The wind is blowing my brother away.
He is going away now:
As if he was just popping out to the shops;
As if he just put the phone down;
As if he went for a walk and just carried on;
As if he got a cold and became cold.

I remember the tale of the Alcoholic who told his wife
He was just slipping out for a packet of cigarettes
And wasn't seen for five years.

My brother is not migrating like a bird
Nor is he folding over the world,
Like the moon,
To grow thin,
Disappear and
Come back new again.
He is not a season you can be sure of,
Eventually.
He is no fairy tale,
For in the story, they live happily ever after.
And in this case, the last four words do not apply.

He doesn't have a writer's block.
There is nothing more to write
And all there is between us are the memories we made.

So shall the days go.

He is dying of Aids.
But who is there to aid him in this death?
A midwife for life...
Who shall bring him out?
Who shall give death to him?
Ease him in his labours,
His dying pains?

Who shall husband him,
Mother to him,
Hold him?
And shall he cry out like a new-born babe?
Cry out against the shortness of his years,
The tight span he squeezed to the last breath,
That ended by squeezing him?

No answers,
For answers only come at the end.
And no-one is going the whole way with him.
It is his death.
He must own it.
He must die it.

And if there is light,
Why is it so full of darkness?
And if there is faith,
Why can I only question?
And if there is peace,
Give him some,
That he may sleep.

A.P.

To My Brother

It has come to this,
Mark.
Your crying cuts me.
How can I reach you?
On the telephone, your voice is
Already that of a ghost,
Soft,
Disjointed your words
As the painkillers try to
Soothe your thoughts.
How can I say
That I shall take the pain away?
I do not presume on God.

Your time is slipping away like oil,
The coloured patterns you made in this life
With one splash
Are gone,
Forgotten.

Death is sweet-talking you,
But your body is so sour.
Death is singing to you now.
Walk with him.

Thrush will take your breath,
Not the singing bird,
But a fungus filling your throat,
Stealing your poet's voice.
It is hard now for you to swallow,
Hard for all of us to swallow.

How you cried to me like a child,
And me a dumb ox,
Saying over and over,
I love you, I love you
As if love were enough.

Your death is a fact
As inevitable as the falling of the sun.
Not one prayer,
Nor a million
Shall keep her in the sky
One second longer than
The gravity of the universe dictates.

And I won't be there when you die,
But will instead be walking the
Hills of our forefathers,
Spilling my tears onto Czech soil.
Let me know the moment,
Let the wind whisper it me
And for a second,
The wheat may bow its head
And mourn with me
As the world is made less by your going.

But can I cry out to the passing people,
Stop what you are doing!
My brother is dead!?
They will shake their heads,
Laugh at my foolishness
And walk on.

How,
If I have said goodbye,
Do I keep saying it over and over?
The bow of your dying
Bent and pulled back
Until it was thought the archer
Could never release his grip
And the arrow find its
Mark.
This time,
It shall not miss.

Miss you,
Brother.
See you.
Love you.

A.P.

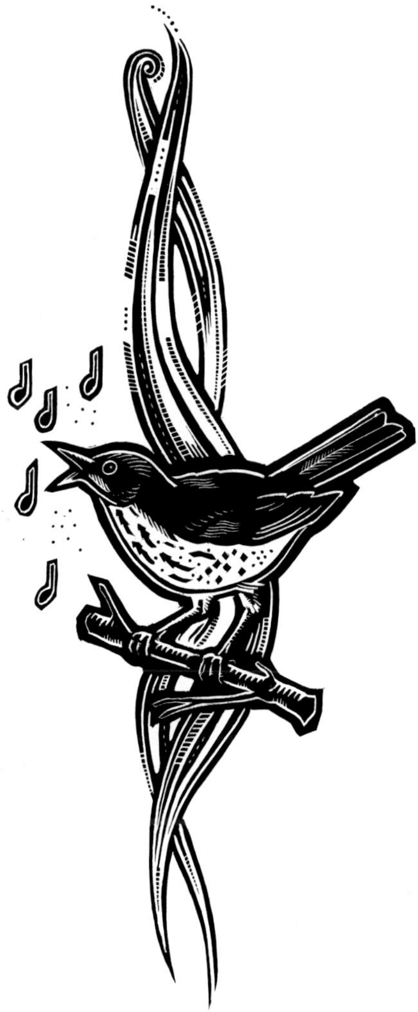

Your Dying Is Such A Mess

Your dying is such a mess!
Said the father,
You can stay in your room,
Until you've tidied it up!

Said the New Age Therapist
And what have you
to learn from death?
As the young man fought
For one more breath.

I have seen so many die,
Muslim, Buddhist, Jew,
And only the Christians seem to be at Peace!
Said the Born Again Nurse,
Matter of fact,
And smothered in fat.

Said the Grandfather,
You're tired! You're ill! It is bad!
And I have got a terrible headache!
Yet then, they prayed together,
In the language of his people.

Said the Bug Exterminator
With fear on his face,
As he stole around
The hooked up, younger-than-him man,
These ants are no big problem, man!

Said the brother,
I have a life,
And a beautiful wife
And you are small and shrivelled.
But in the darkening hours,
How he cried.

Said the boy who was dying,
Help me.

And the friends did not talk,
Only came to
Bring food,
Wash clothes,
Get what was needed,
The necessary prescriptions of love.

A.P.

Last Poem

I call the legions of angels
to be my witness.
I have bared my back
and shovelled steel for centuries
and am now bloodless, wan as dawn.

I offer flesh, my mind,
the sundance,
and then fall with the effort,
this fall,
this cold and freezing fall,
in front of the Capitol
and I am not alone.

The dead thing lies within me,
agitating, fomenting, deceiving, rotting,
and the air's gentle caress
tugs it from its thorny layer,
saying come out and play,
ugly child of mine,
spawn of my fatal loins,
death of all generations,
death of all hope and fecundity.

I shall never bear another son,
and Polly will ripen,
and my brother a proud father
will be.

Yes, this is a Spanish song
I am singing,
I am felled by the brutal bull,
I matador, my knives
and cape not sharp nor
quick enough to stop this beast.

Then mourn then,
mourn for the dust and the blood
that settles on my lips,
cakes my face,
making me that which is not,
yet was once,
me, Mark.
Wail now,
this death is significant.

I am the alpha, the omega
the bloody circle,
the eyes and limbs of the children
of darkness,
and this disease is gospel,
so help me Christ.

When a man seeks a jacket,
give him two,
lead him to a soft water
and comfort him,
and when a woman seeks
a protector,
swathe her in warmth
and give her hope.

The brutality and inconsistency
of this life
is,
and rum and morphine
only serve to close the door awhile,
the darkness claws its way in nonetheless,
so hold her,
and never, ever, let her go,
unless she wishes it,
then do so.

We have much to learn,
the elements in our body
rebel,
too much,
too much
and they want to sleep.

Sleep now , in Grace,
don't bury me.

M.P.

Part Three

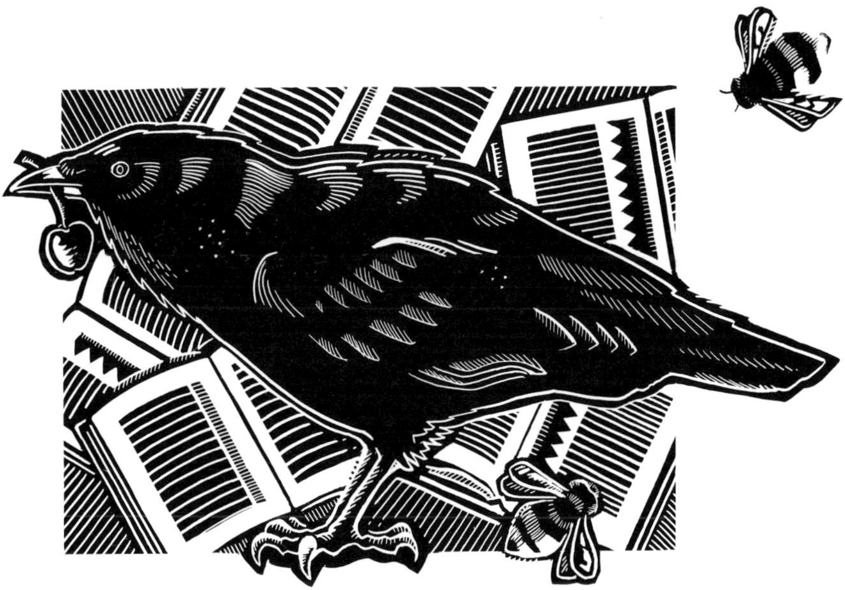

DEATH

Excerpt From The Journey-William's Story

"The war ended there
for some; for those who died;
who went home whole.
Others remained, between jagged alternatives:
the comfort of irresponsibility,
or the egg of fear;
hard, filled with the tortures
of love, hope, care, friendships.
What could a man know when war was his mind?
Violence, his angry God?
Trembling fear always on his lips,
in his heart's deep core.
It is then, that warmth is grief,
the smile a knife.

I stayed to help these ones,
to help men reconcile themselves.
I prayed with them, fed them
with bent spoons by candlelight.
The enemy was always there,
within. The enemy was fear,
fear of life, of death, of love,
of lovelessness, of riches, of poverty,
of families...These men died to save their families,
and lost them.

I watched this kind of death daily,
moving from village to village,
town to town, across borders,
across rivers, wherever I could go.
God, we were limited,
reading scraps of old newspapers
to them, to save their failing sanity;
lying with them till their bodies stopped shaking;
praying with them, great prayers,
the prayers of the dying,
O they were heard before they went.

Can I paint for you,
the colours of this war,
the dark misery,
the violet tragedy
blooming in the bruised brains of men?"

M.P.

When The Boy Died

When the boy died,
he had not eaten for two weeks.
Cotton soaked in the juice of lemons
had been pressed to his lips
to moisten them.
His breathing bed had
stretched him out
until he was almost bone -
thin enough then for the
eye of a needle.

It was morning
and the year turned in circles,
summer shivering and growing cold,
winter uneasy in sleep.
Someone was looking for him,
and he was tired of running.
Wouldn't it be nice to lay me down in sweet waters....
he thought, parched and oh! so thirsty.
The time was close now,
to put away his things and go.

A tear squeezed out of the spring of his eye,
running in a tiny river down his face.
This was the body's last sadness for itself.

And then he stood up.

It was a miracle of death,
a true Lazarus,
that moment he slipped from his skin like a fish.
He sat himself down by the door
and waited.
He had stayed this long,
a few more pieces of time would not weigh him down.
And they came,
the loved ones,
and ah! their tears were greater than tiny rivers.
They were bees,
clustered around the honey of his body.

I am here! he whispered,
and though they could not hear,
the words were a warmth
to sweeten the cup of their tears.

Came the mother then,
called in the early morning,
running,
gasping,
heavy like labour
with the birth of such new and wailing grief.

I am here! he whispered,
and she knew for a second, peace;
turned to the door,
puzzled
frowning,
remembering something important.

How could he soothe her now?.....
I am here! he whispered,
and somehow the silent words gave comforts,
a life buoy thrown from one dead,
helping her not to drown.

Now all his words,
his allotted words were done.
He looked with slowness around the little room,
to all that he was -
crystal, picture, book, the cloth of his body;
all no longer needed nor necessary.

A friend was calling him
in a voice familiar as dreams.
Time to go,
to leave the room of his house,
the four small walls of his days.
Outside, the trees were singing to him,
leaf songs,
elegies of wind,
as he stepped out,
cradling his death
like a lullaby.

A.P.

On Seeing My Brother's Body Lying In His Bed

Bright was the sun-lidded thirteenth August day you died.
My mother prayed to close your looking eyes, could not
Stop the way they stared askew. Gasping, she tried
To fit the face with one she knew. Then, she
Cried. For this still life can never hide
The deal your illness made. You lost,
Much more than a pound of flesh,
Breath for bone, skin to hide,
Perfect skeleton
With arms of string,
What knots have
You un-
Tied?

A.P.

The Silent Days

These are the silent days.
Men are walking slowly by,
departing in trains,
arriving at destinations,
leaning on iron railings.

These are the silent days.
The silence of laughter
moving through the ribcage
of the mind,
so many faces,
too many faces,
the laugh is in all of them...

the laugh that leads to life,
to suicide,
the tide that brings birth,
bears death,
that washes up the pilgrim,
the harlot,
the child, the dead,
the laugh that leads here,

here being the silent days
where gods are walking
with hands in their pockets,
too idle to dice,
too slow to make miracles,
too dull to care...
the cards are falling
randomly.

These are the silent days.
A small wind enters my house,
water falls on leaves,
water falls on stone,
the sound of seasons, cycles, systems,
the whole thing going round.

These are the silent days.

M.P.

For Mark

For when my brother dies,
I shall cry tears of stone.
Never will I have felt so alone
And my heart will try to be hard.

For when my brother dies,
No more late night Monopoly and after
Bacon and eggs with a cup of laughter,
The yolk of dawn just breaking.

For when my brother dies,
I shall cry a city of tears,
Then put on a smile, hide all my fears
If only I could, if only.

For when my brother dies,
No more hate and family spite,
Now I'm fine, everything's all right,
But I will miss the making up.

For when my brother dies,
I shall cry blades of grass.
People will be polite, dare not ask
Why my garden overgrows.

For when my brother dies,
I shall have no brother,
No other to hug and to hold
And I the younger,
Am the one who will grow old.

A.P.

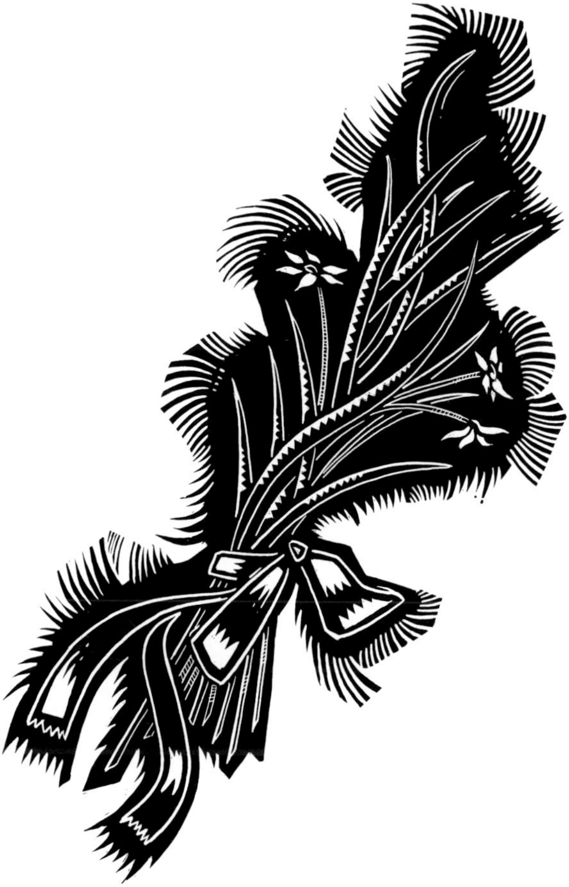

The Grief Box - A Sonnet

I'll fit you into verse with skillful ease,
Politely asked, mime the right words to say -
Be strong! Carry on! It's all in a day!
Tie up each feeling, the English Disease,
Ignore my heart as it grieves, as it grieves.
Soon, a smile, like the moon comes, shining ray,
My friends shout out *Onwards we go!* as they
Ignore my heart and it grieves, and it grieves.

But there comes a time, I just cannot contain
It, this stone, hell-heaviness of my tears
Now brims, burns me to bear this bastard pain
I did not ask for, and it is so plain
You were not planned like rhyme. Then, what is clear,
My brother lies dead, this poem in vain.

A.P.

The Advertisement

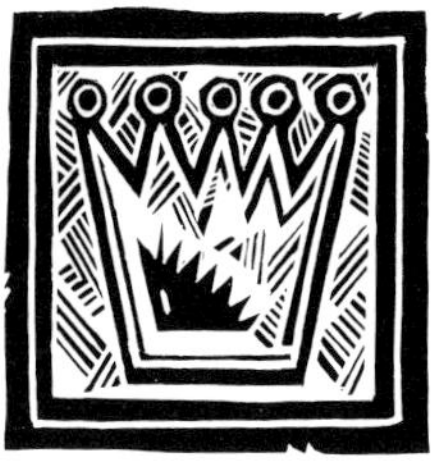

Benetton, Benetton
Where have you been?
Ah! We have been
To see the dead queen

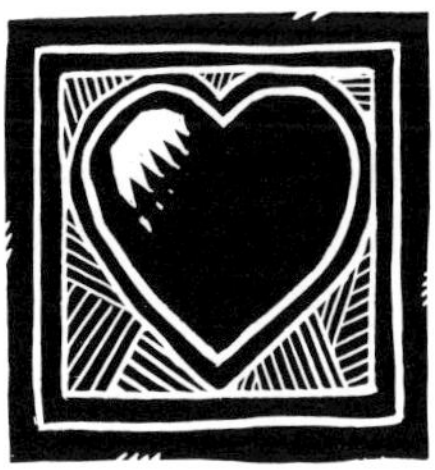

Benetton, Benetton,
What found you there?
We found some money
To be made for the fair.

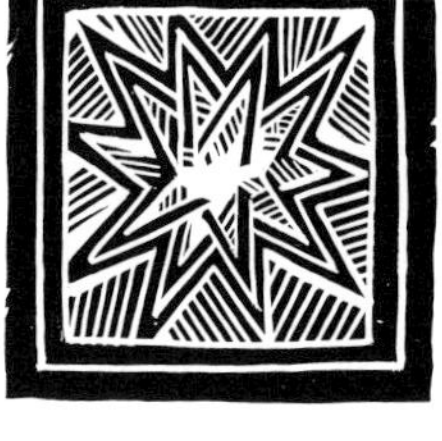

Benetton, Benetton
What did you then?
We took him up front
Again and Again
And Again and Again

A.P.

I Have Become Most Intimate With Death

I have become most intimate with death
of late.
He has opened the door of my house three times.
Strange, that he came to visit,
stranger still, the door swings out
and those that are close,
one by one,
have left.

I have become most intimate with death
these last few years.
Easy to call him a common thief, but
when it comes to the case of my brother
I would prefer cat-burgling as a metaphor -
The man who stole my brother's breath from right under his nose!
We have all kept silent about it since.
Even if his breath was recovered,
It would only be wind.

I have become most intimate with death
these last few months.
How he plucked the jewel of our baby
from my wife's womb,
God only knows.
When we received the news,
our security system burst into fear.

I have become most intimate with death
these last few days.
My grandmother of eighty-six years
was ripe and ready for unravelling.
She was as thin as the eye of a needle
and her mind forever losing the thread of memory.
death was a quiet bargain, a snip,
the price she paid to sleep, to dream,
unwind and rest at last.

I have become most intimate with death
too late.
Like some huge accordion player,
he is squeezing out my years.
The door swings out in perfect key
and I must sing along, pray
that my life may be of some note, to someone,
when tomorrow becomes today.

A.P.

Washington DC, Spring 1994

Another spring day has begun in Washington DC.
Bright the sky and the trees
filled with the food of
a thousand little winds.

I am sitting in your room,
the big white wide room you slept in,
the room you ran the family business from,
the room you were engaged in,
the room I was so jealous of,
with its view across the park.....

before the illness came and made you small,
and you could not fit in such a spacious space anymore.
It had outgrown you,
And we, the family, had to move you
into another house,
with meaner rooms.
No stairs to hinder you now,
as all your walking had been done.
I still find it odd
that you, the vital man, are dead.
For your things surround me here,
the key ring my mother carries is yours,
though you are turning keys in different doors;
your car sits in the street,
waiting for you to step out of the house,
reverse this present into the past,
now that would be an amazing manoeuvre.

They have put your things in a cupboard,
to be sorted and sieved,
but no-one can put away the places that we shared,
street corners we met on,
hills we tobogganed down,
pavements we ran along,
sun we sat under,
all this would be so hard to fold away
in the back of my mind,
and so shall I always take these places with me,
for there is room in the yardstick of my heart.

A.P.

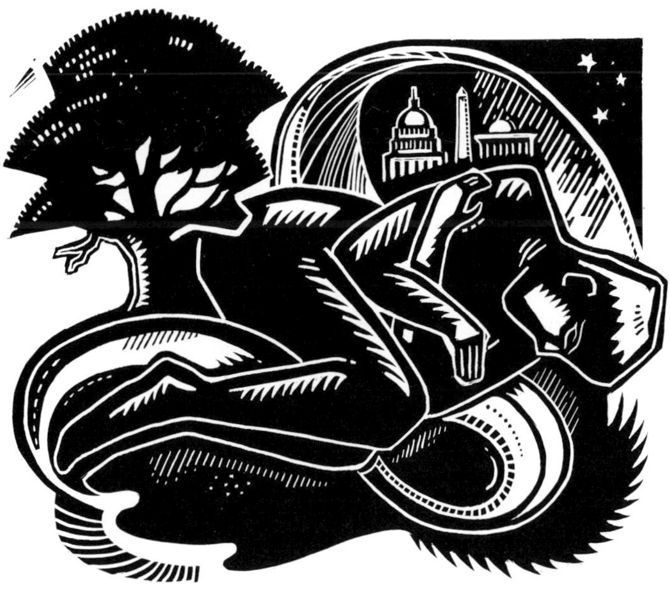

I've Been So Clumsy Since You've Gone

I've been so clumsy since you've gone
Plates just jump, then shatter on
The floor, all that matters fallen
Away. I am in pieces with it all.

Each time I reach out with my hand,
Cups slip through my fingers like sand:
Time has passed, and our set of six
Is one less. Love, nor glue can ever fix

What was, nor craftsman replace your
Thin and fragile life, restoring
You to me. Aids broke your body,
Left only sharp, jagged memory.

A.P.

Part Four

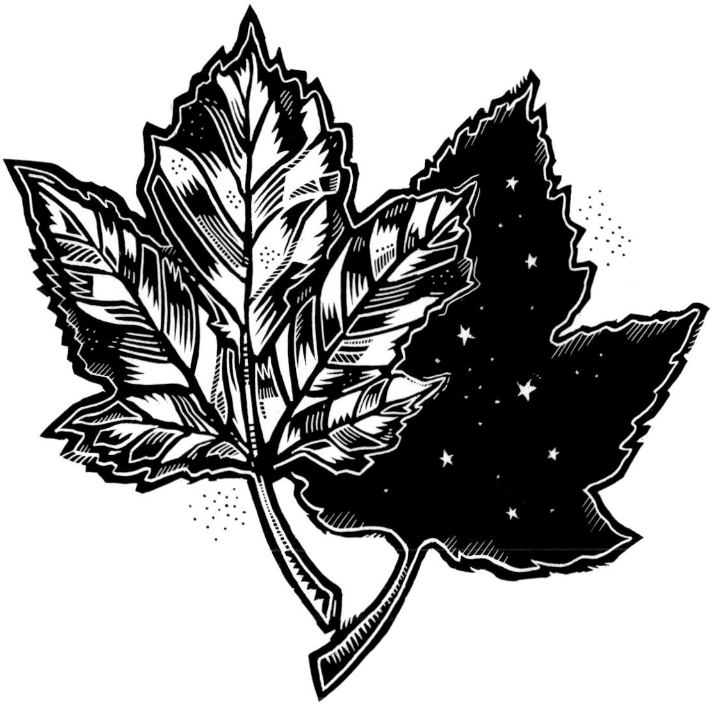

REFLECTIONS

That's All

Think of this,
dream.
We may be close,
as close as air
or blood or earth
are.
We are one
by nature
of all nature.
What we give
or lose
is not given,
lost,
just is.
Your brilliant eyes
now,
my words
now
are,
that's all.

M.P.

That's All

I think of you,
dream,
am closer now,
as close as touch
or thought or breath
were.
We have won:
despite death,
all of death,
what we lived
or loved
was not left,
lost,
just was.
Your blazing words
flow,
my crying eyes
flow
far,
that's all.

A.P.

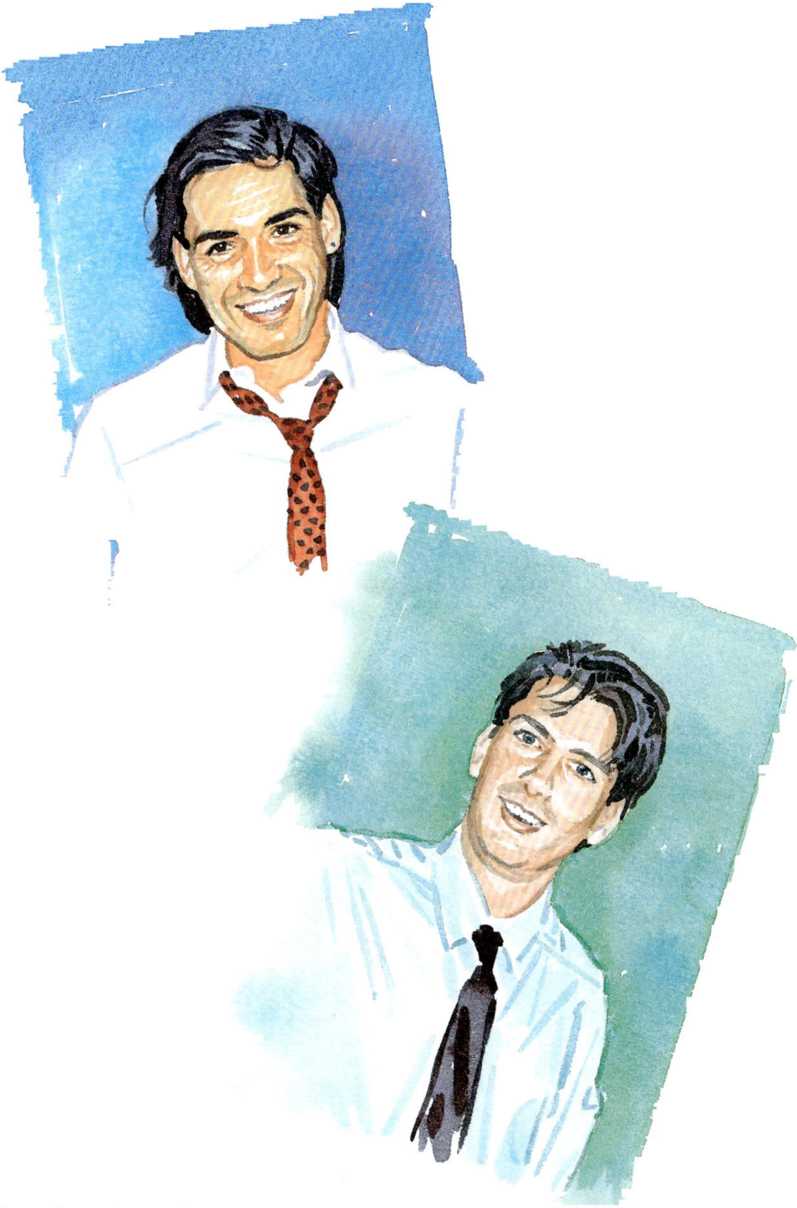

Mark and Andrew Peters

Michael Ogden

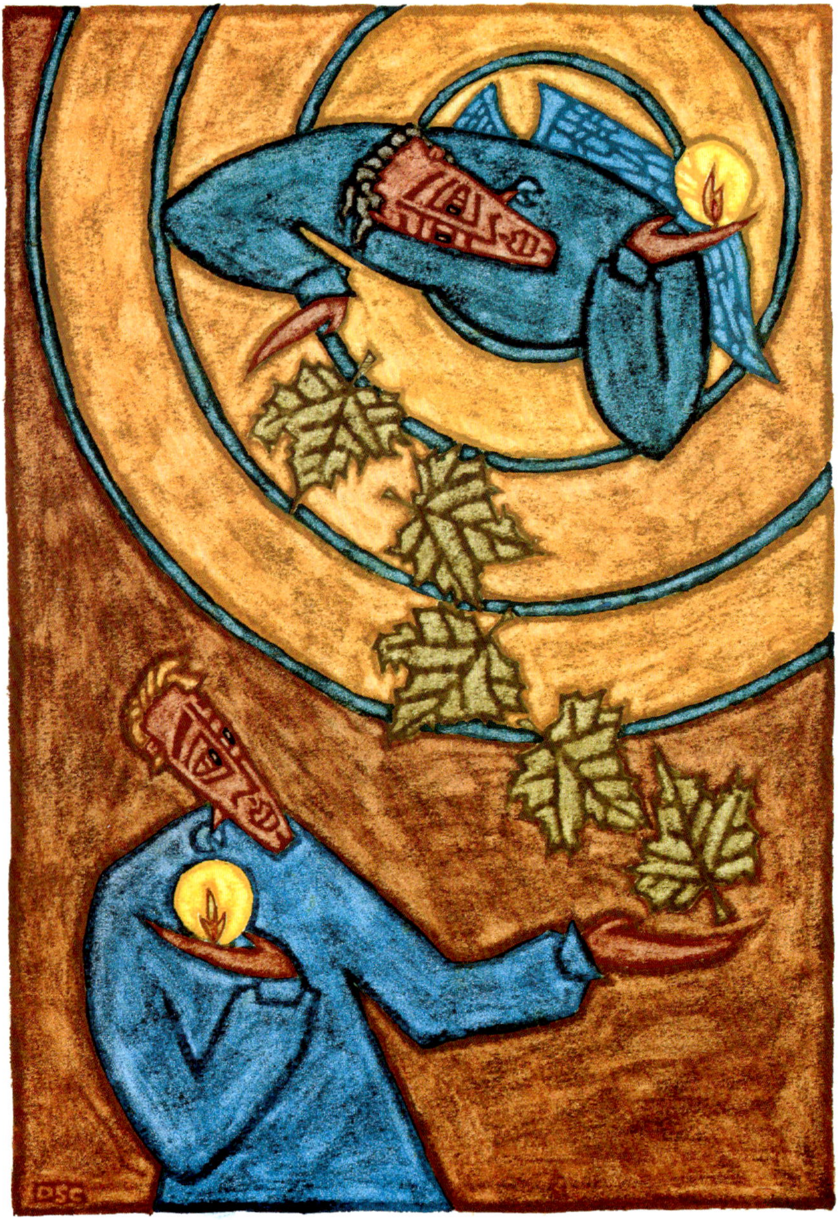

Council a Human

Dianne Cartwright

No More Than This

I am no more than mud,
yes mud and dust,
red blood red mud red clay,
my bones are in the
bottom of the creek,
I am no more than
bone and water,
mud, blood and life.

I want no more than rain
and salt,
I am no more than what
I want,
rain and salt, blood and dirt
are that,
and that alone.

And Nature
in my blood is love
and dirt, and dust, and water,
in my love is salt
and rain,
I am no more than blood
and water,
dust and love,
no more than this.

M.P.

Words

I am words that have not been said,
I am a book thrown against a wall,
left to curl and yellow by a fire's edge ...
O yes, I am words,
words that wrap around me
like a lover's arms,
lie dangling with a voltage
fit to raise the dead.
Words not yet spoken
drift within the daylight,
the darkness,
and I am so tired tonight.

One short life,
this ...
Owen, Keats,
the elder statesman Yeats,
the Eliot I will never be.
Just words.
and left to me is
this:
to die quiet,
a small print,
a small patch
to lie forgotten,
but in the corners
of my brother's heart.

M.P.

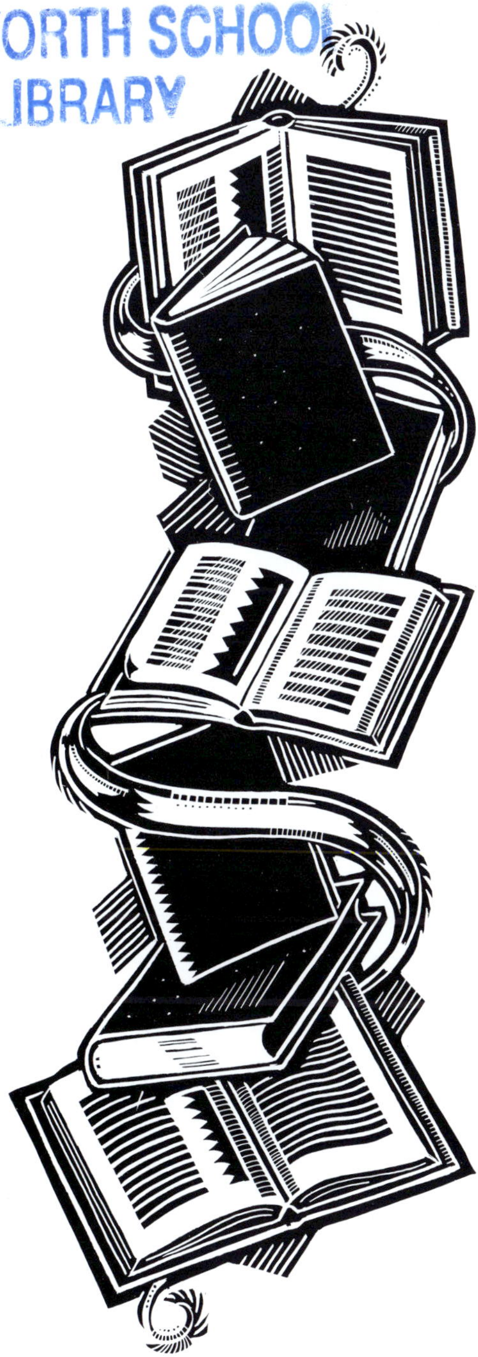

Poem

A poem rests in the wind,
rests in the footprints
of the earliest horse,
runs through the palm fronds,
the sucking marsh,
the beauty and terror
of electricity, gases,
intelligent acids.

A poem like the ash and dust
that our great poets are,
a countless ream
of silvered scripts,
the sound of stones,
water,
fire,
gas.

Standing here
before a rock that
bears the prints
of animals three million years ago,
bears the prints of things
repeated,
the poem continues still.

M.P.

This Great This

See how they tumble and glide,
see how they fall and rise,
see how their wings fold and glisten,
see how their faces glow, O listen
to the music, O listen
to childhood and adulthood ...
see how we are born,
seeds in the orange sun,
seeds in the black dung,
seeds in the hard places,
seeds in the softest niches,
see how we are born ...
all feet and eyes,
tears, fluids, and breath,
fire and fire only;

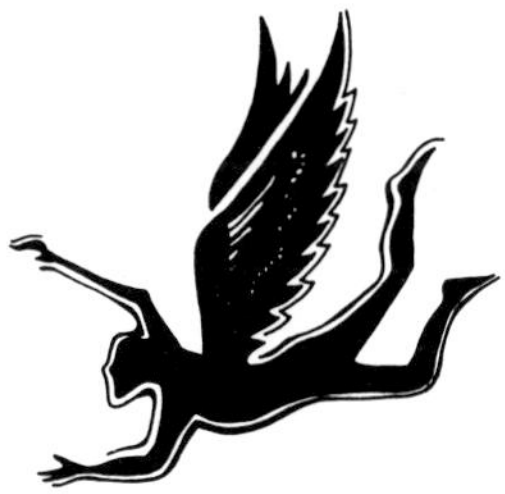

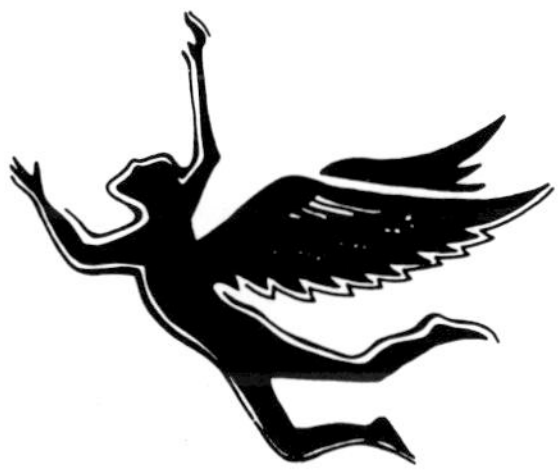

how the sounds of angels,
how the sound of children,
how the sounds of animals,
of child-gods
turn this time into spirals
of celestial information,
stringing light, sound, smell,
touch, taste, it and this,
that and that
into this,
into this Great This.

M.P.

The Anniversary

My dearest brother,
A year has fallen since you left,
Whirling my world around
Like pods of Sycamore.

Today,
Comes Old Friend Grief
With her knotted hands,
and me,
A tangled ball of string,
Unravelling days of stretched out sorrow.

Closer she beckons,
Womanly Grief
With her begging bowl of tears,
And if I let her in,
And if I let her through my door,
Will she sing to me songs,
Give to me small comforts?

The tears come like sudden guests,
Unasked,
Unanswerable,
Ladled out in good measure by
Old Friend Grief.

It has taken one whole year
To gather in our sheaves of words.
Their ripeness is all,
But I alone
Am eating the fruit.

There is an emptiness inside
Success,
Nor love,
Nor making of love
Can crack
This endless rounded o.

My hollowness a bag
And Old Friend Grief
The ancient bag-lady
Shuffling through the years
And the prayers
And the layers
And the tears.

A.P.

I Shall Make You A Poem Brother

I shall make you a poem brother
Each thought fine as thread
But will it sow up
Your heart
Your heart?

I shall make you a poem brother,
Then lay it gently on your head
A lullaby to close
Your eyes
Your eyes

I shall make you a poem brother
With words as warm as my hands
To wrap you up and
Hold you
Hold you

I shall make you a poem brother
Unlike me it shall be strong
A strong box of words to
Bury you
Bury you

I shall make you a poem brother
And it will be filled with earth
Soft blanket of soil to
Cover you
Cover you

I shall make you a poem brother
Mould every sentence into a seed
Then sprinkle them quietly onto
Your bed
Your bed

I shall make you a poem brother
And if one of the seeds that fell should grow
Only then can I let
You go
You go

Fine
Lullaby
Warm
Words
Filled
Quietly
Grow

Each thought
Lay it gently
With words
Unlike me
And it will
Mould every sentence
And if one

Your heart
Your eyes
Hold you
Bury you
Cover you
Your bed
You go

A.P.

Scattering the Ashes

Ah! you have gone and all that is left is words
that ring like dull bells on my tongue
and my mouth is dry
as the ashes of your body.
For one whole year
and a month,
we held you in a plastic bag,
airtight - for there was no longer any need to breathe.
And you sat in the living room of our mother's house,
squat, monolithic in your black-cornered container.

Easy to say the spirit had gone,
jumping out from your body as the last breath exhaled.
Yet in those clustered granules
were hands I held,
rough scraping chin,
your gangly angularities,
the dark eyes I begin to forget.

And so we took you, my brother,
up onto the hill,
with scissors and bags and hands,
ready to dip into you,
the bitterest sherbet.

We found an avenue of trees,
a lane of childish days
where women with dogs avoided us,
the weeping mother,
the cold-eyed son
unable to comprehend the vastness of his grief.
We scooped you up
to place you at the beginning of each trunk,
an offering, a grey sacrifice,
and for a second,
as my hands grew powdered
I wondered with horror
if that which killed you,
lived still in this sickened chalk.

And my mother, laden with the years,
the endless avenue of deaths which she had had to walk,
fell to the grass and cried out
at this ancient and greek tragedy,
on the hill that myth said was made by bodies from the plague.

We stumbled home to finish the job
of spreading my brother out
in the places we best remembered,
and in the garden
I gathered my handfuls
and sowed at last my tears,
One for the wasp's nest,
One for the pear tree,
One for the feast,
One for the fire,
One for the den, and
One for the cut down willow,
where we played the perfect game of hide and seek.

You are hidden now,
cut down in the maleness of your days.
We have buried the last of you
by the roots of a young and eager silver birch.
My mother is made grey by your ashes
and your terrible gift to me
is an oldness in my youth
and a fear of death
that cannot see the life growing inside my wife's womb.
This is a dark day,
I would, if I could now put it away,
to scatter its shadows
among the many-memoried summers we shared.

A.P.

The Year Is Falling Now

The year is falling now, but so unlike
The ending of this year, you shall not come
Again. The Ash tree curls her fingers tight
Against the cold, for she still holds a spark
Of sap, but you, my brother Mark, are gone;
Your body burned to ashes cold and still;
So cold, how small this box of memory,
All that there was of my brother, now dark.

All that there was of my brother, a spark
So bright, it flamed like a radiance.
How many were touched by the Mark
You made. You made your entrance
And it was bold and bright:
Mark me! Man of Wealth!
Quick Mind! Good Sight!
Rude of Health!
Diamond
Sharp
You shone
Out like fire,
Until spirit
Began to tire
Your brother, the poet,
Did not want to let you go,
Nor see this body's burning spark
Grow thin as embers losing their glow,
All that there was of my brother, now dark,

Dark like leaves falling to an endless sea,
Carried curling from this bright body's barque
In waves now rough, now soft to rock you gently.
What can be carried with you? What bright thing?
Your watch? Your purse? Quick mind? Smile of rich pursed lips?
In death, there is no room for carrying
On, nor time, and all that was simply slips
Away, leaving me to carry the leaves
Of poetry you wrote with fingers curled.
My heart is falling now, though it believes
A wind of words might blow you from this world.

And you at last have made your perfect Mark
On paper, this ship of breath, this bright ark.

A.P.

Part Five

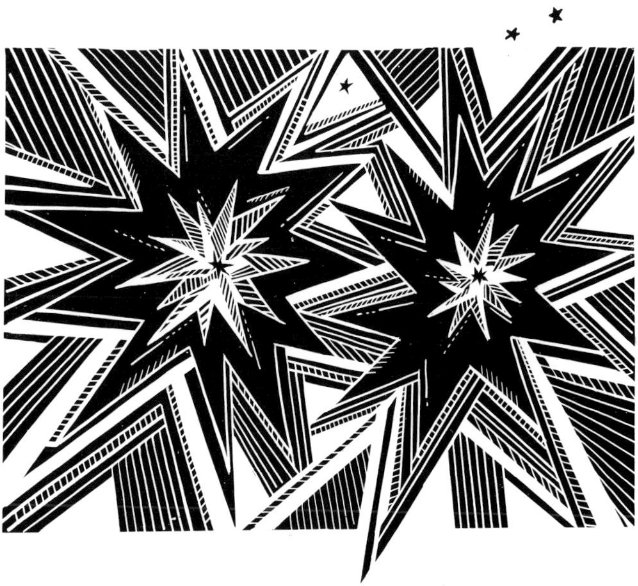

RESOLUTION

Counsel A Human

Counsel a human on transience,
counsel this being on death,
on life,
on the flowers and minerals,
the cities that spring from the rocks,
O counsel them.

Counsel them with a soft word,
song like bird song,
sound like cornwind,
mother murmering to life within.
O counsel them.

Grandfather, grandmother,
father, mother,
brother, sister,
partner,
waiting for life, for death,
to spread like flame blankets,
oil burning on water,
waiting for the fragile
burnt ash of an autumn leaf
to settle in form,
melt in the wind.

M.P.

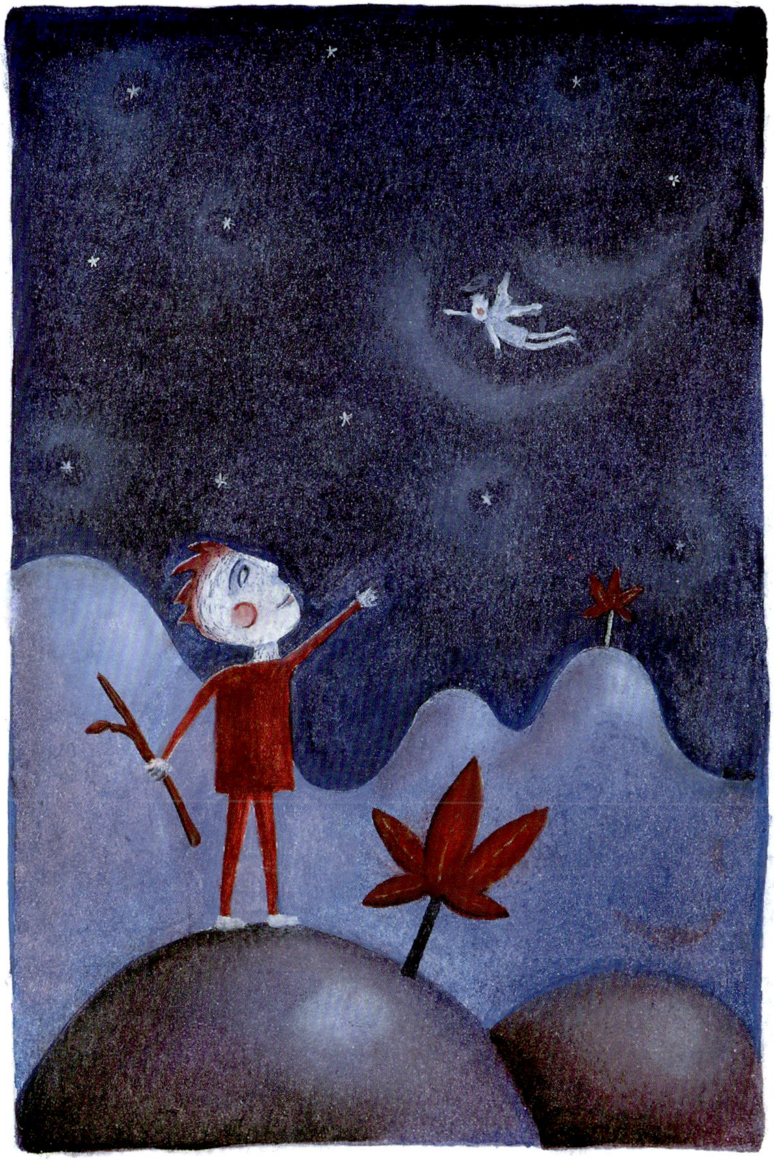

The Wayfarer's Charm

Liz Marshall

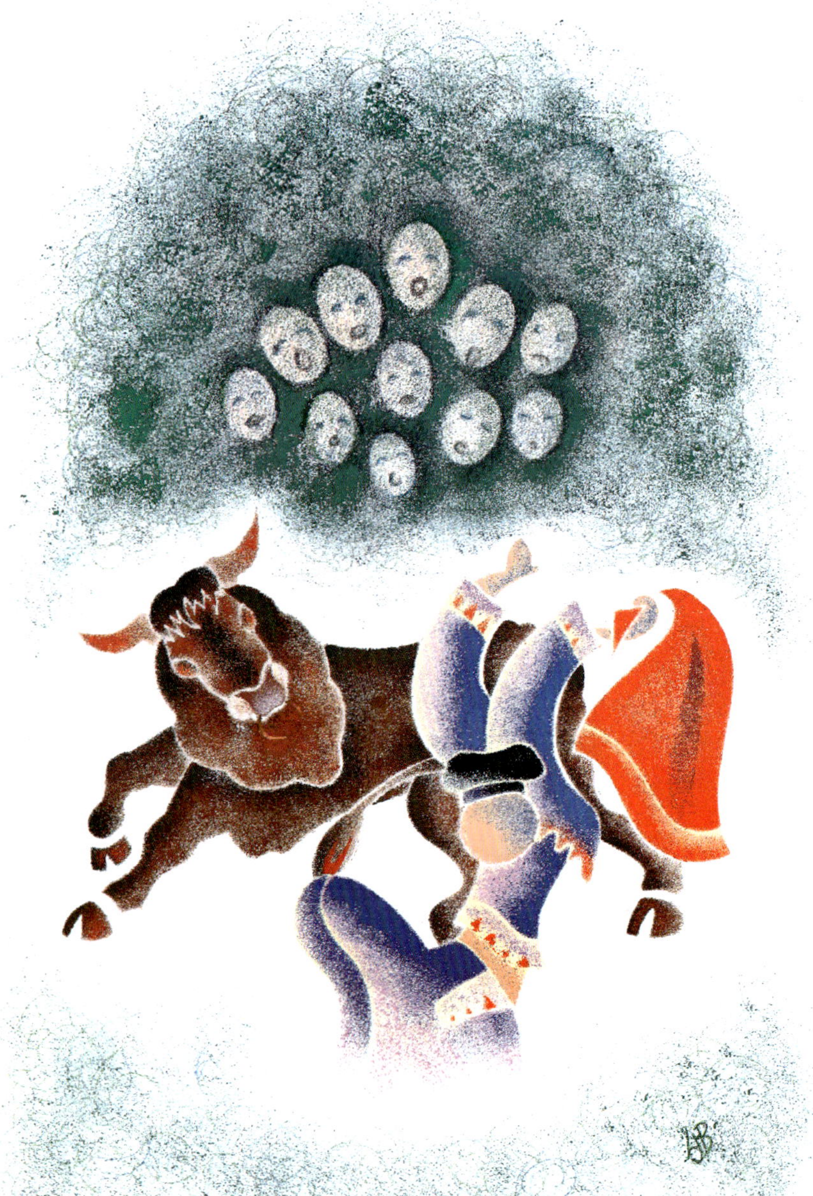

Last Poem

Lorna Bond

Life with him was sometimes living hell.
Yet in the end, I loved him well
And got my revenge with a little villanelle!

Well, you might think I'm funny in the head
But my brother popped by the other day
Which was quite odd, considering he's dead.

In his life, he wanted to be known, well read
And though he's now a bit short of breath, it's OK,
Well you might think I'm funny in the head.

The promise of posthumous fame and all that cred
Brought him back. A little ego goes a long, long way.
Well, you might think he's funny in the head,

Only he hasn't got one, and when all is said
And done, he has a spirit's sense of play.
Well, he might think it's only fun ahead.

Yet who shall do his signings, who his groupies bed?
But that's what brothers are for, I say
Which is quite right, considering he's dead!

The book is out, and maybe we shall be Laureatéd,
And he is shouting silently Hip! Hip! Hooray!
Well, you might think I'm funny in the head,
But he's quite glad, considering he's dead!

A.P

Hyaa!

My brother's heartbeat is a drumbeat

hyaa! hyaa!

a love song sung along a web
of lines,
one for your sister,
one for your ancestor,
one for the fire breathing,
tube-playing circle.

My brother's heartbeat is a pattern
in the dust,

hyaa! hyaa!

with one eye closed
and the other rolling high,
from miles away they
can hear the velvet-skinned
painted man play.

My brother's heartbeat is a note
upon the winds,

hyaa! hyaa!

women's loins quiver
young boys shiver
nodding elders raise
their eyes,
the lines far and wide
are shaking to the sound.

My brother's heartbeat is the final sound,
that's it,

hyaa! hyaa!

the thick turgid rumble,
the quiet mouse soprano,
the love note,
the sound that makes the heart kick,
the heart start,
that wakes the people into wonder.

hyaa! hyaa!

M.P.

Pursue The Light

When all light melds into
a muted tapestry,
a beautiful, deep horizon
where one thing is ever less
distinguished
from the next,
how can I struggle to preserve
my drowning form,
carbon to carbon?

Not to pursue the light
is work indeed,
the faint light at the
door of death,
the large light at the
gate of life.
Light is mirrored on the
water,
so why do I laugh,
looking up beneath?

M.P.

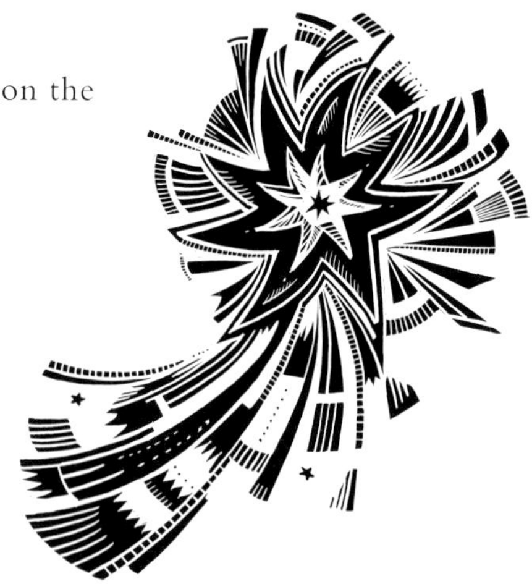

January

I feel you are so far away from me now,
As if you had moved into a room in my house
That is no longer there.

When I was young, I dreamed
Of London landscapes that
were always just beyond
what I knew so well by day:
streets had new turnings,
mountains soared behind familiar hills.
I dreamed these places
over and over
until they became a part of me.

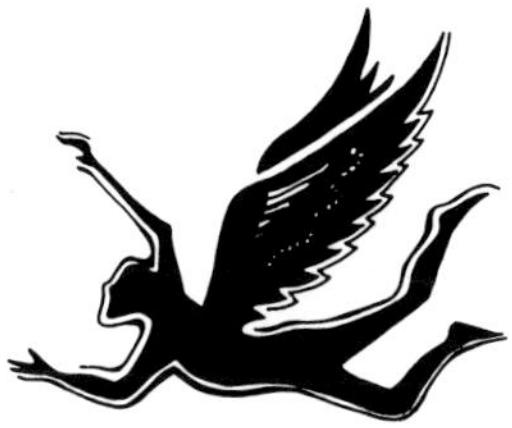

I wake up,
and you are not there,
nor can I even feel you anymore.
I need photographs to
remind me of your face,
for you are blurring at my edges.

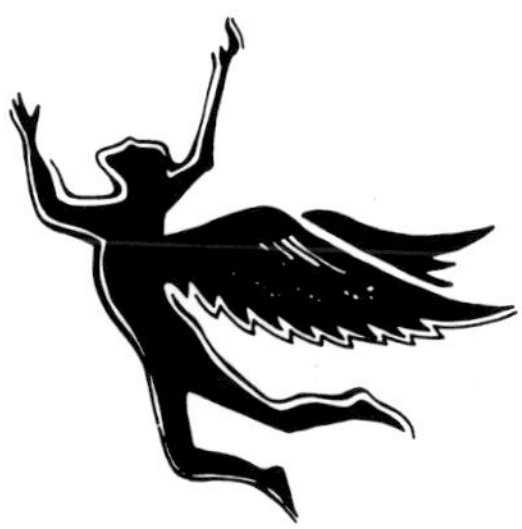

When you first died,
your presence was so palpable.
Sometimes, I would be driving in my car,
and there you were!
right next to me
in the seat,
slap-bang
in that moment
with your crazy smile
and leather jacket
I was always jealous of.

It was a thumbs-up to my life,
the brotherly encouragement
I always craved.
And you had to finally die
to give me this gift.

Now the year
is new.
You stayed for but a little while,
bowed by family,
hovering, uncertain,
like an angel,
maybe checking up on little brother
and that he was OK.

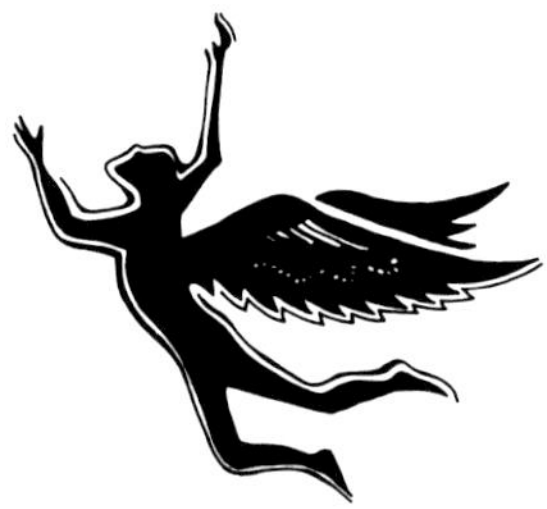

The year moves on
and you too have ways to go.
I do not know them
and try as hard as I can,
cannot see,
only feel
the lengthening distance
between us.

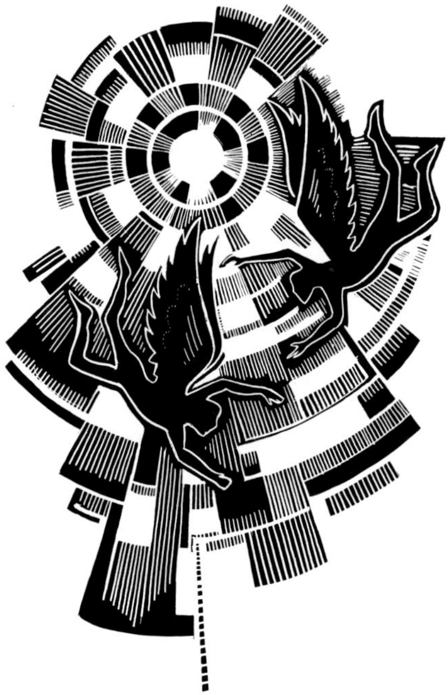

Again,
we have to say goodbye
and if you get
this letter of letters,
let me know
how you are keeping.

And now?
And now you are falling away
as these words do.
God speed, brother
and may the angels be with you.

A.P.

Seal Our Hearts

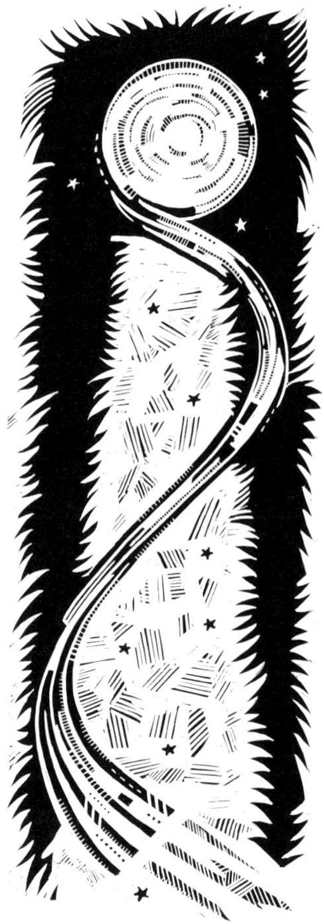

A ladder is descending
from the moon,
and if these feet could walk,
they would,
and if these feet could walk,
they would;

A ladder is descending,
a white trail to the edge of time;
time waits now for a foot to step
onto the water's surface,
the path is straight
and all the moment asks
is walk.

Walk to the circle of light,
the broadening cone-center,
the moon's radius,
light-limbed,
light-spirited.

I take a step
from land to sea,
the sea's womb rises
to honour me,
and my thoughts scatter, making music
like so many prehistoric stones,
milling and singing in the surf.

I hear your voice in the waves ...

Seal my heart:
East-West, North-South,

I feel your touch in the stars ...

Seal our world:
East-West, North-South,

I know your presence in the azure night ...

Seal our house:
East-West, North-South,

and the moon gently is
as large as our being.

M.P.

The Wayfarer's Charm

May every road that leaps
to greet you
be blessed with a wayfarer's charm,
may the forests and valleys,
mountain passes and hilltops
be blessed with still, small voices,
for the way is long
and the comforts required,
day by day,
step by step.

Give thanks to the angel
that's walking with you,
the little child
whose innocence lights
the every place,
the small and gentle animal
wrapped around your feet,
the gentlest tug and pull
of wind,
the touch of light,
the warm caress of dark,
secure sleep.
May the angels be with us.

M.P

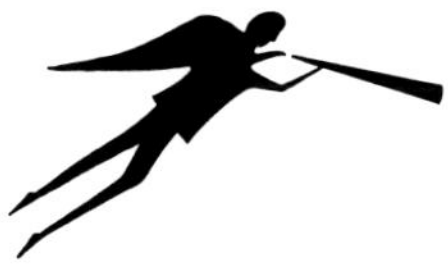

Biographies

Andrew Peters

born 2nd July 1965

It was whilst reading English at Corpus Christi College, Oxford, that Andrew Peters discovered his one true love in life: words. He began to direct and perform in poetry shows and became poetry editor of ISIS (The Oxford University Magazine.)

During the mid to late Eighties, Andrew established himself as part of the performance poetry collective Angels of Fire, appearing at such gatherings as the *Avon Poetry Festival* and the *London Festival of Performance Poetry* at the Riverside Studios in London. He began to make a living running poetry workshops, adult education classes, poetry residencies and In-Service training in schools.

National recognition was achieved in the nineties with regular invitations to appear at the *BBC Poetry Festival for Children* and the *Cheltenham Festival of Literature.* His work has been recorded several times for Radio 4's *Talking Poetry* and other appearances include *Blue Peter*, *The Big Breakfast* and *Anderson Country*. Publications include poems in various anthologies, the most recent of which is *The Poetry Joke Book (Macmillan)*, and he has a collection of children's poetry *Word-Whys* (*Sherbourne*). *Salt is Sweeter than Gold* (an adaptation of a Czech fable)is published in Britain and the US with *Barefoot Books* and *Shambhala.* 1995 sees the publication of his *Barefoot Book of Strange and Spooky Stories.* His AIDS poems have appeared in *Heart Throb* (the West Midlands Arts literature magazine) and the national AIDS anthology *Jugular Defences* (The Oscars Press).

Mark Edward Peters

Born 25 May 1961. Died August 13 1993

Mark Peters spent most of his late teens fighting drug addiction until he moved to start a new life with his maternal Czech grandparents in Washington DC. Winning the battle against drug addiction, he also won a scholarship to the American University. He studied Literature and Comparative Religion, meanwhile editing and writing for the university magazine, *American Literary*. His poems were also accepted for publication two years running in the *Allegheny Review, (The National Journal of Undergraduate Literature.)* His poetry also won a special award and was published in the *American Collegiate Poet's Anthology (International Publications)*.

A major figure in the Washington literary scene, Mark took part in and produced a series of poetry festivals and was published in several national journals. On graduating *Cum Laude*, he became assistant editor and contributor to *New Realities*, a national arts and philosophy magazine. In 1989 he was engaged to be married and preparing to begin a Master's degree when he was diagnosed HIV positive. Although his academic career was cut short, Mark continued to work and set up a network and library on HIV related issues.

His first collection of poetry *Angel Parade* was published on the 11th August 1993.

Index

A Child's Poem *A.P.* *20*

Autumn Spirits *M.P.* *30*

A Time of Year *M.P.* *32*

Child Song *M.P.* *19*

Counsel a Human *M.P.* *86*

Excerpt from The Journey - *William's Story* *M.P.* *50*

For Mark *A.P.* *58*

Guy Fawkes Night, Primrose Hill *A.P.* *12*

High up in the Hills *A.P.* *38*

Horse of Night *M.P.* *34*

Hyaa! *M.P.* *90*

I Have Become Most Intimate With Death *A.P.* *62*

I Shall Make You a Poem Brother *A.P.* *78*

It all Happens Here *M.P.* *14*

I've Been so Clumsy Since You've Gone *A.P.* *66*

January *A.P.* *93*

Last Poem *M.P.* *46*

Life With him was Sometimes Living Hell.... *A.P.* *89*

My Brother's Snoring *A.P.* *13*

My Soft Heartbeat *M.P.* *25*

No More Than This *M.P.* *71*

On Seeing my Brother's Body Lying in his Bed *A.P.* *55*

Poem *M.P.* *74*

Pursue the Light *M.P.* *92*

Scattering the Ashes *A.P.* *80*

Seal Our Hearts *M.P.* *96*

That's All *M.P.* 68
That's All *A.P.* 68
The Advertisement *A.P.* 61
The Anniversary *A.P.* 76
The Burning of Stubble *M.P.* 16
The Dance is Begun *M.P.* 37
The Fair on Hampstead Heath *M.P.* 9
The Flame *M.P.* 24
The Gift *A.P.* 8
The Grief Box - A Sonnet *A.P.* 60
The Illness *M.P.* 31
The Seed (For my Father) *M.P.* 26
The Silent Days *M.P.* 56
The Wayfarer's Charm *M.P.* 98
The Year is Falling Now *A.P.* 83
To my Brother *A.P.* 40
This Great This *M.P.* 75
Washington DC, Spring 1993 *A.P.* 22
Washington DC, Spring 1994 *A.P.* 64
When the Boy Died *A.P.* 52
Words *M.P.* 72
Your Dying is Such a Mess *A.P.* 44

'May the Angels be with us' was produced with the help of the following:

Graphic Design:

Legend Design,
33, Eastfield Road,
Westbury on Trym,
Bristol BS9 4AE
Telephone 0117 9621333

Colour Illustrations:

Adrian Barclay	*'Autumn Spirits', page 35*
Lorna Bond	*'Last Poem', page 88*
Dianne Cartwright	*'The Fair on Hampstead Heath', page 18*
	'Counsel a Human', page 70
Liz Marshall	*'The Illness', page 36*
	'The Wayfarer's Charm', page 87
Michael Ogden	*'Guy Fawkes Night, Primrose Hill', page 17*
	Andrew and Mark Peters, page 69

Black and White Illustrations:

Josephine Sumner

Printed in England by Westernprint Limited, Wiltshire.